Ultimate Dementia Activities For Seniors

Eazy bizzy to unlock joyful moments: Step by step Guide to Empowering adults and Alzheimer patients…

By

Mildred Kent

TABLE OF CONTENT

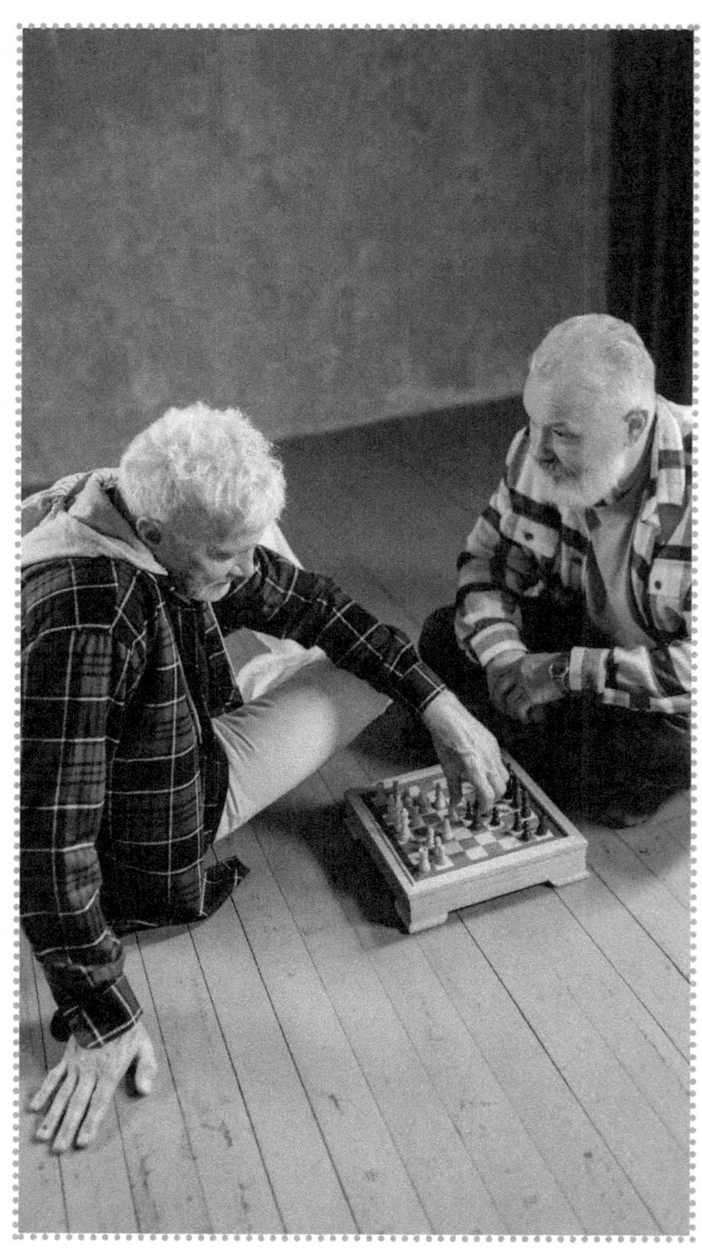

CHAPTER ONE

INTRODUCTION

Previously, the focus on identifying a person's cognitive and functional deficits overshadowed their subjective experience of living with dementia, which was based on a biomedical model based on symptoms and neurological explanations (Hubbard et al. 2003). Since it was believed that information from those who were actually affected by the disease was unreliable due to their cognitive and functional decline, information from proxies—both informal and professional caregivers—was frequently used to understand people with dementia (van der Roest et al. 2007). (Aggarwal et al. 2003). Over time, a shift occurred, and individuals with mild-to-moderate dementia have described their subjective experiences of living with dementia in a large body of research (Gilmour & Huntington 2005, Langdon et al. 2007, Preston et al. 2007, Parsons-Suhl et al. 2008). Hearing about the lives of those affected by dementia is crucial to comprehending their subjective experience and preserving their identity.

Background

Research reveals that individuals suffering from dementia attempt to strike a balance between developing new aspects of themselves and preserving their identity while adapting to the disease's effects on their lives (Holst & Hallberg 2003, Steeman et al. 2007, MacRae 2008, Beard et al. 2009). According to Caddell and Clare (2011), this indicates that the participants are experiencing both continuity and change in their sense of self at the same time, placing them in a state of flux. This is true even in the early stages of the illness, since research has demonstrated that individuals with severe dementia can still have a sense of self and identity (Tappen et al. 1999, Beard 2004).

A social constructionist theory that emphasizes the significance of language can help us understand how crucial it is for dementia patients to preserve their sense of self. The structure of ideas and experiences, and consequently the formation of social reality, can be influenced by language proficiency (Gergen 1985). The story of our life and the various social identities we create in collaboration with others are integral parts of our sense of self and the concept of selfhood, which are strongly related to personal identity (Harre & Gillett 1994). (Sabat & Harré 1992, Sabat & Collins 1999). The identity itself is told as a narrative with distinct locations, scenes, characters, storylines, and themes.

Life stories are psychological constructs that are jointly created by the individuals and the cultural setting in which their lives are situated and given significance. Certain memories are chosen and interpreted by individuals as self-defining, giving them a higher place in their life narrative than others. In light of this procedure, identification might be viewed as a chosen outcome. Individuals select the experiences they believe have shaped who they are and given their lives meaning and purpose (McAdams 2001).

A life story needs to meet two requirements, according to Linde (1993). A life tale should first contain a few evaluative elements that convey the narrator's moral principles. Second, the events in a life story should hold a particular significance for the narrator, enough that they can be told and retold for the rest of their lives. Self-stories, according to Polkinghorne (1996), are a means of giving people's lives a cohesive identity by compiling their prior deeds and experiences into an insightful narrative. The life tales cover information from the time of a person's birth to the present and beyond. People are always living their life story, and those who are suffering from dementia are no different.

Though occurrences in the future may alter the significance of some past events and their perceptions of how the remainder of their lives will unfold, what has happened to them in the past cannot be altered. Life narrative work is a popular intervention in the treatment of individuals with dementia and is seen as a crucial component of person-centered care. To preserve identity and a sense of self among persons with dementia, the work can be defined as a means of gathering important components of a person's past and present and should be viewed as a continuous activity rather than a one-time event (McKeown et al. 2006). Family members frequently gather life tales from those who have dementia (Subramaniam et al. 2014). And is typically chronicled in a life story book that contains written narratives about significant life events, photos, and the individual's experiences and accomplishments (Webster & Fels 2013).

Given that dementia can impair language (American Psychiatric Association 2000), it is preferable to begin life narrative work early in the disease, when individuals are still able to tell their own story (Clarke et al. 2003, Meininger 2005). Dementia patients may have trouble speaking, following, and taking part in complicated conversations with others (Warchol 2006, Hydén & Örulv 2009). Furthermore, they may exhibit erratic awareness and attention, as well as concentration lapses (Downs 2005). People with dementia may find it difficult to recount their life experience when they get to the point when their language and concentration are impaired. Allowing individuals who are in the early stages of the illness to tell their own story is crucial because it makes it more likely that their own life narrative will be reflected rather than the narrative as family members or caregivers have understood it. In person-centered support, this is even more crucial. Having a deeper understanding of the way individuals living with dementia see themselves and their lives increases the likelihood of supporting them in continuing to lead fulfilling lives.

1. Being Aware of Dementia

Although the phrases dementia and Alzheimer's disease are sometimes used synonymously, they refer to two distinct illnesses. A broad spectrum of symptoms that impair an individual's capacity to carry out daily tasks on their own are collectively referred to as dementia. The most prevalent and well-known type of dementia is Alzheimer's disease. It is a gradual illness that deteriorates with time.

Dementia symptoms and indicators

Certain dementia symptoms can be reversed, depending on the underlying cause, of which there are numerous. While memory loss is a common symptom of dementia, it does not indicate the presence of dementia on its own. Some medical illnesses that can be treated can have symptoms similar to dementia.

Dementia symptoms include:

- Modifications in cognitive abilities
- alterations in language and conduct
- Reduction in memory Reduction in focus and attentiveness
- inadequate decision-making and reasoning abilities

indications and manifestations of Alzheimer illness

While dementia is a general term, Alzheimer's disease is one specific kind of brain disease. It is characterized by dementia symptoms that worsen over time. Early indications of Alzheimer's disease frequently include problems in memory, thinking, and reasoning abilities since the disease initially affects the area of the brain linked to learning. The signs of the illness worsen with time and include disorientation, altered behavior, and other difficulties.

Alzheimer's disease's early warning signals include:

- Mood swings, including despair or other alterations in behavior and personality
- Disorientation about time or place
- inability to focus, plan, or solve problems
- Having problems with vision or space, such as misplacing objects, getting lost, or not recognizing distance when driving
- Language issues, such as difficulty finding words or a limited vocabulary while speaking or writing Memory difficulties, such as trouble recalling specific incidents
- difficulties with everyday tasks, such writing or using dining utensils, at work or at home
- Making poor judgments
- avoiding social or professional gatherings

identifying Alzheimer's disease and dementia

It can be difficult to diagnose dementia and determine its type. Your healthcare team will assess the individual's abilities by looking at the pattern of their loss of function and skills.

In order to diagnose Alzheimer's disease, patients must self-report their symptoms and take tests to evaluate their ability to think and remember. Even though this can be challenging, a number of diagnostic techniques can assist in identifying dementia and determining, with a fair amount of accuracy, if Alzheimer's disease or another illness is the cause.

Addressing Alzheimer's and dementia

The majority of dementias and Alzheimer's diseases have no known cure, but symptoms can be managed. Drugs can aid in the treatment of memory problems and other cognitive disorders.
People who have been diagnosed with dementia or Alzheimer's disease should be ready for changes in their condition as they occur since these conditions can be unpredictable and progress gradually.
Among the strategies to improve the wellbeing of an individual suffering from dementia or Alzheimer's disease are:
- ensuring that they are getting enough food
- promoting consistent exercise
- checking the individual's hearing
- Keeping them engaged in social events

2. Importance of Activities for Seniors with Dementia

The importance of meaningful and interesting activities cannot be emphasized in the context of dementia care, where the complexity of cognitive decline and memory loss loom large. Activities catered to the needs and abilities of seniors and elders suffering from dementia are vital resources for improving their quality of life, promoting emotional stability, and maintaining cognitive function. This thorough investigation delves into the profound importance of activities for elderly individuals suffering from dementia, revealing the many advantages that go beyond simple stimulation and include social interaction, emotional connection, and a feeling of identity and purpose.

Understanding Dementia [A Complex Landscape]

Dementia poses a significant challenge to both the affected person and their caregivers, as it is typified by a decline in cognitive function that goes beyond what is typically associated with aging. Different types of dementia, such as Alzheimer's disease, vascular dementia, Lewy body dementia, and others, show symptoms in different ways. Symptoms can range from confusion and memory loss to behavioral and personality changes. People with dementia struggle with a loss of autonomy, a deteriorating sense of self, and an increasing reliance on others for care and support within this complex web of cognitive decline.

Activities' Effects on Cognitive Function

Purposeful activities can act as a beacon of clarity amidst the fog of forgetfulness and confusion that accompany dementia, stimulating neural pathways and maintaining cognitive function. According to research, mentally demanding activities like word games, puzzles, and reminiscence therapy can help delay the onset of dementia-related symptoms and slow down cognitive decline. These activities enhance cognitive reserve by stimulating the brain and promoting neuroplasticity, enabling people to sustain higher levels of cognitive function for extended periods of time.

Emotional Well-being [Nurturing the Heart and Soul]

Activities are essential for maintaining emotional health and giving dementia patients a sense of community and connection, even outside the domain of cognitive improvement. The emotional toll that dementia takes, which is marked by depressive, anxious, and frustrated feelings, emphasizes how crucial it is to provide chances for happiness, participation, and deep conversation. Research has demonstrated that engaging in music therapy, art therapy, and sensory stimulation activities can elicit positive emotions, alleviate stress, and improve the general quality of life for individuals suffering from dementia.

Social-Engagement-[The Power of Connection]

Social activities, whether in group settings or one-on-one interactions, can mitigate feelings of loneliness and isolation, foster meaningful relationships, and promote a sense of community and belonging. Among the group activities that dementia patients can participate in are singing groups, exercise classes, and reminiscence circles. Social isolation is a significant concern in the field of dementia care, with individuals experiencing a shrinking social network and a diminishing sense of connection to the world around them.

Well-being [Caring for the Body]

Physical activity plays a critical role in maintaining general health and well-being, even though cognitive function and emotional stability are frequently the main focuses of dementia care. Exercise on a regular basis that is customized for each person's ability level strengthens muscles, lowers the risk of falls, increases functional abilities, and improves cardiovascular health. Physical activities tailored to the needs of seniors with dementia offer a holistic approach to wellness, addressing the interconnection of mind, body, and spirit. These activities range from gentle stretching exercises to outdoor walks and chair-based workouts.

Identity and Mission [Respecting the Person]

An essential component of person-centered dementia care is acknowledging the distinct identity, life experiences, and preferences of every individual. Engaging in activities that draw from an individual's interests, pastimes, and history honors their uniqueness and keeps them feeling like themselves. Activities that align with a person's identity and values, whether through familiar hobbies, significant rituals, or nostalgic reflection on past experiences, offer a sense of fulfillment and purpose, confirming their inherent value and dignity.

Making-Memories: [A Comprehensive Approach to Care]

Activities are the threads that connect happy, meaningful, and meaningful moments in the lives of people with dementia, creating a tapestry of care. Through adopting a comprehensive approach to care, which includes mental stimulation, emotional stability, social interaction, physical well-being, and a feeling of self and purpose, caregivers can establish settings that support the full person, significantly and meaningfully enhancing their lives.

Final Thought: Engaging People to Empower Their Lives

The value of activities for seniors and elders in the dementia care process cannot be emphasized. Activities play a critical role in improving the quality of life for people with dementia, from preserving a sense of identity and purpose to promoting social connection, supporting emotional well-being, and stimulating cognitive function. Caregivers can empower individuals to live meaningful and fulfilling lives while upholding their dignity and improving their journey through the intricacies of dementia by embracing the power of engagement.

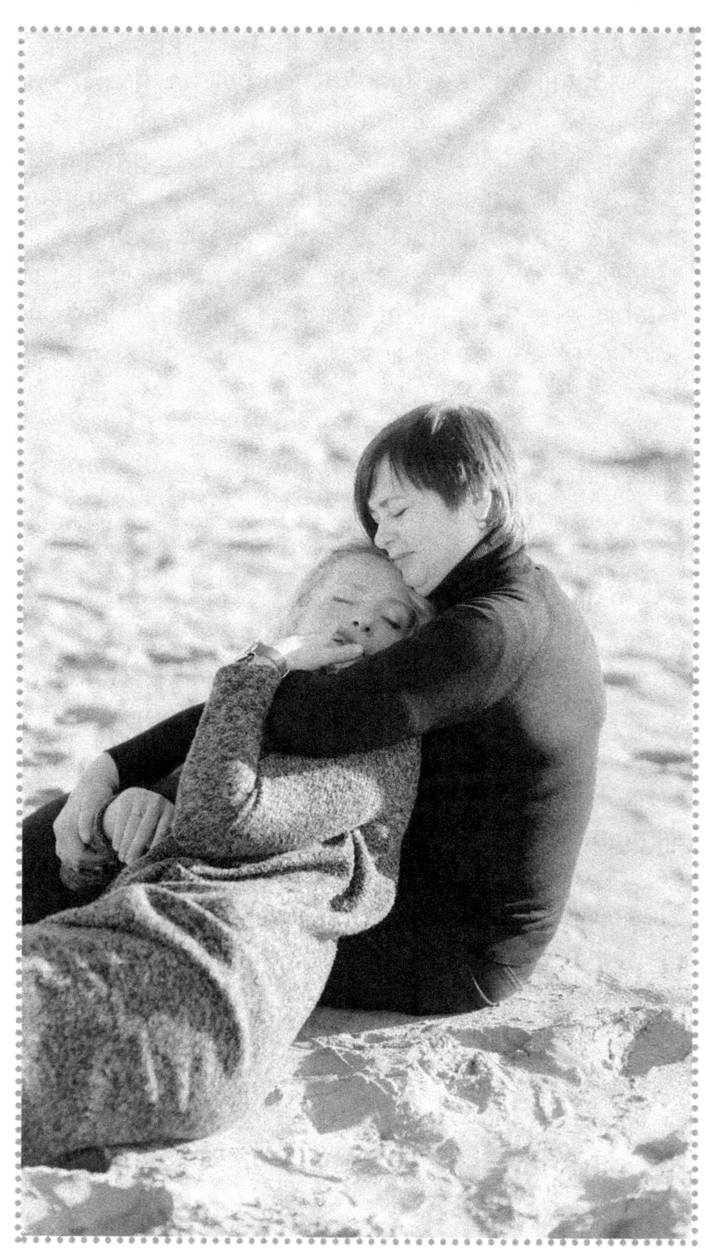

CHAPTER TWO

Setting the Stage for Engagement

Creating an Enriching Environment for Patients with Dementia

First of all,
There are unique difficulties that arise when providing care for a loved one who has dementia, especially when it comes to encouraging participation and preserving quality of life. People suffering from dementia may become more withdrawn or uninterested in their surroundings as their cognitive abilities deteriorate. However, carers can significantly improve the wellbeing of dementia patients by establishing an environment that is stimulating to the senses, evokes memories, and encourages social interaction. This guide aims to provide dementia patients with strategies for creating an environment that encourages engagement and makes them feel more fulfilled, connected, and stimulated.

Recognizing Dementia

The most common cause of dementia is Alzheimer's disease, which is followed by Lewy body dementia, vascular dementia, and other types. Dementia frequently manifests as memory loss, communication difficulties, poor judgment, and behavioral or emotional changes. each with a unique set of signs and a distinct course. Common dementia symptoms that interfere with speech include:

1. **Memory Loss**: People with dementia frequently have trouble remembering names, dates, and specifics, which makes it difficult for them to carry on meaningful conversations.

2. **Language Impairment**: As the illness worsens, people may develop aphasia, have trouble pronouncing words correctly, or have trouble understanding spoken language.

3. **Disorientation**: People with dementia may experience disorientation, which makes it difficult for them to focus or follow conversations.

4. **Behavioral Changes**: Mood fluctuations, agitation, and frustration can make communication even more difficult, necessitating caregivers to be patient and understanding.

Establishing-Helpful Environment

The physical surroundings greatly influences how people with dementia perceive their experiences. Adapting a home or care facility to the special needs of dementia patients is part of creating a supportive environment. A few things to think about are:

1. **Safety**: To avoid falls, remove any potential hazards like loose rugs or electrical cords. To improve safety, install handrails on stairs and grab bars in bathrooms.

2. **Familiarity**: Fill the person's environment with recognizable items, pictures, and keepsakes that bring back pleasant memories and comforting sentiments. Establishing a memory area adorned with artifacts from their history can offer a feeling of consistency and safety.

3. **Clear Signage**: To assist people in independently navigating their surroundings, use labels and signage that are clear. Clearly label cabinets, drawers, and rooms with legible text to cut down on confusion and annoyance.

4. **Natural Light**: Get as much natural light as possible as it can enhance mood and help control sleep-wake cycles. During the day, keep the

curtains or blinds open and, if you can, think about putting in more windows or skylights.

5. **Calming Elements**: Use components like calming hues, cozy furnishings, and décor with a natural theme to encourage rest and lessen anxiety. To create a relaxing atmosphere, try turning on some soothing music or natural sounds.

6. **Clear Layout**: Making living areas accessible and well-organized can help lessen confusion and annoyance in those suffering from dementia. Individuals can become more independent in navigating their surroundings by using visual markers, color-coded cues, and clear signage.

7. **Personalization**: Adding cherished memories and familiar items to a dementia patient's living environment can help them feel more like they belong and help them develop a sense of identity. Having a space that is uniquely yours can improve sentiments of familiarity and comfort while fostering wellbeing.

Using Your Senses

Providing people with dementia with sensory stimulation can be a very effective way to keep them engaged and improve their general wellbeing. In order to foster engagement and connection, caregivers can design meaningful experiences that stimulate the senses of sight, hearing, touch, smell, and taste. To stimulate the senses, try these methods:

1. **Sight**: To draw attention and create visual interest, put bright textiles, flowers, or artwork on display. To improve visibility and make objects stand out, use contrasting colors.

2. **Hearing**: To arouse memories and encourage relaxation, play well-known music or songs from the person's past. To have a customized listening experience, think about utilizing headphones or earbuds.

3. **Touch**: To stimulate the sense of touch, provide tactile activities like hand massages, textured materials, or sensory toys. Provide opportunities for soft plush toys or gentle pet therapy with a lovable animal.

4. **Smell**: Create pleasing scents that can evoke happy memories and feelings by using scented candles, essential oils, or freshly baked goods.

Steer clear of overpowering or potent smells that could be uncomfortable.

5. **Taste**: Considering any dietary constraints or sensory sensitivity, provide snacks or drinks that suit the person's taste preferences. Encourage people to socialize by having meals or snacks together.

# 1.	Encouragement-of-Social Engagement:

For people with dementia, social interaction is crucial to preserving their emotional stability, cognitive abilities, and sense of self. Caregivers have the ability to promote social interaction by offering chances for meaningful interaction with peers, family, friends, and other caregivers. The following tactics can be used to encourage social interaction:

1. **Family Visits**: Welcome frequent visits from loved ones and family members, who can offer company, consolation, and opportunities for reflection. Arrange multigenerational events like storytelling, art projects, or family dinners.

2. **Group Activities**: Plan leisure events and activities that promote social engagement and interaction. Think about engaging in activities where people can share memories and experiences, like music therapy sessions, group exercise classes, or reminiscence groups.

3. **Volunteer Opportunities**: Offer dementia sufferers volunteer opportunities that provide them a feeling of direction and a way to give back to the community. Opportunities for volunteer work could include simple tasks or projects assistance, animal therapy, or gardening.

4. **Intergenerational Programs**: Collaborate with nearby educational institutions, childcare facilities, or neighborhood associations to organize intergenerational events that unite people of all ages. Mutual learning and meaningful connections can be fostered through intergenerational activities like music performances, art projects, and reading buddies.

5. **One-on-One Interactions**: Regular visits from family members, volunteers, or trained staff can help prevent feelings of loneliness and foster a sense of connection by offering personalized attention and companionship. Individuals suffering from dementia can have meaningful conversations and activities catered to their interests and preferences when they interact one-on-one.

6. **Support Groups**: Leading support groups for family members and caregivers can help them deal with the difficulties of taking care of a loved one who has dementia by providing them with a sense of camaraderie, practical guidance, and emotional support. Support groups can lessen caregivers' feelings of loneliness and burnout by offering a platform for exchanging experiences, coping mechanisms, and resources.

Keeping Up a Routine:

For those suffering from dementia, routine and structure can offer a sense of security and predictability, which helps to lessen their confusion and anxiety. A daily routine makes things easier to manage and more pleasurable by fostering a sense of purpose and order. The following advice can help you stick to a routine:

1. **Maintain a Consistent Schedule**: To give your day structure and regularity, set aside specific times for meals, activities, and relaxation. Make visual calendars or schedules to assist people in anticipating and getting ready for upcoming events.

2. **Simplify Tasks**: To lessen overwhelm and frustration, divide tasks and activities into tiny, doable steps. As necessary, provide verbal cues

and prompts to help people through each step of the activity.

3. **Flexibility**: Adjust and change as necessary to meet evolving needs and preferences. Let people take part in activities at their own speed and in their own way, adapting as necessary to suit their interests and abilities.

4. **Balance**: To avoid exhaustion and burnout, create a healthy balance between scheduled activities and unscheduled relaxation. Create opportunities for people to unwind and rest so they can refuel in between activities.

5. **Meaningful Engagement**: Draw from the person's interests, pastimes, and past experiences to design activities that are relevant and meaningful to them personally. Adapt activities to their skills and interests in order to give them a feeling of direction and success.

For those suffering from dementia, creating an enriching environment calls for careful planning, imagination, and compassion. Caregivers can improve the quality of life and general wellbeing of dementia patients by creating an environment that encourages engagement through sensory stimulation, social interaction, routine, and meaningful activities. Caregivers can make the lives of those with dementia more fulfilling by fostering moments of joy, connection, and fulfillment through patience, flexibility, and a thorough understanding of each person's specific needs.

In a nutshell carers can foster a loving and supportive environment that upholds the dignity, autonomy, and sense of belonging of people with dementia by establishing the conditions for engagement. In spite of the difficulties posed by dementia, caregivers can improve the quality of life for patients with dementia by providing sensory stimulation, routine, social interaction, and meaningful activities. Caregivers can significantly improve the lives of individuals with dementia by providing them with moments of purpose, meaning, and connection through their commitment to person-centered care, empathy, and dedication.

Sensory Stimulation

Using sensory stimulation to arouse positive emotions in people suffering from dementia can be a very effective strategy. Sensory activities stimulate the senses of taste, smell, touch, sound, and sight and can arouse memories, calm anxiety, and encourage relaxation. Among the methods for stimulating the senses are:

1. **Music therapy**: Even in the later stages of dementia, music can evoke memories and emotions in those who are affected by it. For those suffering from dementia, playing music they are familiar with or offering opportunities for singing, dancing, and instrument playing can be a source of comfort and enjoyment.

2. **Aromatherapy**: Using fragrances and aromas to create a peaceful and comforting atmosphere can assist in lowering agitation and anxiety in dementia patients. Among the aromas that are frequently used in aromatherapy to encourage relaxation and elevate mood are lavender, citrus, and peppermint.

3. **Tactile Activities**: Giving people with dementia tactile stimulation via hand massages, textured objects, and sensory boards can help them engage their senses and make a connection to their environment. Engaging in tactile activities can help you unwind, de-stress, and feel safe and secure.

4. **Visual Stimulation**: Adding vibrant artwork, scenic views of the outdoors, and visually captivating displays to spaces can pique the interest and stimulate people suffering from dementia. Clutter and an abundance of visual stimuli, on the other hand, should be avoided as they can be overwhelming for those suffering from dementia.

Emotional Support:

The general health and well-being of people suffering from dementia are strongly correlated with their emotional health. People suffering from dementia may feel more understood, appreciated, and respected if they receive emotional support and validation. Among the techniques for providing emotional support are:

1. **Validation therapy**: Although a person's feelings and experiences may appear illogical or confusing, acknowledging and validating them can help lessen distress and foster a sense of security and acceptance. Empathy, respect, and understanding are key components of validation therapy when interacting and communicating with dementia patients.

2. **Empathy and Compassion**: Relieving anxiety and fostering emotional well-being can be achieved by exhibiting empathy and compassion for people with dementia, recognizing their feelings, and providing comfort and reassurance. In order to make people with dementia feel appreciated and respected, caregivers and staff should make an effort to create a warm, compassionate, and understanding atmosphere.

3. **Meaningful Activities**: Giving dementia patients personal, meaningful activities to participate in can give them a feeling of fulfillment and purpose. Engaging in meaningful activities, such as baking, gardening, or religious or cultural rituals, can strengthen one's sense of self and community. To encourage engagement and enjoyment, caregivers and staff should make an effort to include activities that fit the interests, preferences, and abilities of people with dementia.

4. **Person-Centered Care**: This method of providing care entails identifying each person with dementia's particular needs, preferences, and strengths and adjusting care interventions in accordance with those needs. Person-centered care fosters a sense of agency and self-worth by placing an emphasis on the individual's autonomy, dignity, and well-being. In order to help people with dementia feel appreciated, respected, and understood, caregivers and staff members should make an effort to provide a supportive and empowering environment.

2. **Powerful Communication Techniques**

[Increasing Understanding and Connection]

Human interaction is fundamentally based on communication, which allows us to express our needs, wants, and thoughts. However, because of language impairment and cognitive decline, communication can become difficult for those who are suffering from dementia. Dementia is a progressive neurological disorder that impairs thinking, memory, and behavior. Patients with dementia have trouble expressing their thoughts, and caregivers have trouble understanding them. Still, it is possible to have meaningful conversations with dementia patients and improve their quality of life while preserving important relationships with their loved ones.

Successful-Communication Techniques:

1. **Use Simple Language**: Keep your language simple and steer clear of long words or complicated sentences. Talk slowly and in brief, unambiguous

sentences to give the patient enough time to assimilate the information.

2. **Keep Eye Contact and Your Face Expressions Correct:** Nonverbal clues are very important in communication. To communicate warmth, empathy, and understanding, keep your eyes open and make expressive facial expressions. Making the patient feel at ease and appreciated can be achieved in large part with a comforting smile.

3. **Engage in Active Listening**: Pay close attention to the words, emotions, and tone that the patient is using. Even if you don't entirely get their point of view, acknowledge their emotions and validate their experiences. This facilitates the development of rapport and trust, creating a positive atmosphere for communication.

4. **Promote Involvement**: Start a dialogue with the patient by posing open-ended questions and soliciting their opinions. Let them speak at their own pace and refrain from controlling the conversation or interrupting them.

5. **Provide Visual Aids**: To enhance spoken communication, use visual cues like images, gestures, or objects. For example, display pictures

of loved ones or well-known locations to jog memories and encourage dialogue.

6. **Establish Routine**: For dementia patients, predictability and consistency can help lessen confusion and anxiety. A feeling of stability and security can be created by establishing a daily routine and utilizing well-known communication techniques.

7. **Reduce Distractions**: Establish a peaceful, cozy setting for conversation that is free from outside disturbances like loud noises or conflicting conversations. To improve the patient's comprehension and focus, turn down the background noise while keeping your attention on them.

8. **Be Flexible and Patient**: When speaking with individuals who are suffering from dementia, patience is essential. Prepare yourself to restate details, rephrase inquiries, or patiently await answers without losing patience. As you engage with the patient, adjust your communication style to suit their needs and abilities while being accommodating and understanding.

9. **Apply Positive Reinforcement**: Regardless of the result, give the patient credit for their communication efforts. Positive reinforcement motivates patients to continue taking part in

conversations by fostering engagement and boosting their confidence.

10. **Seek Professional Support**: For advice on efficient communication techniques catered to the patient's particular requirements, speak with medical specialists such as speech therapists or dementia specialists. They can provide insightful advice and helpful tools to help the patient and caregiver deal with communication difficulties.

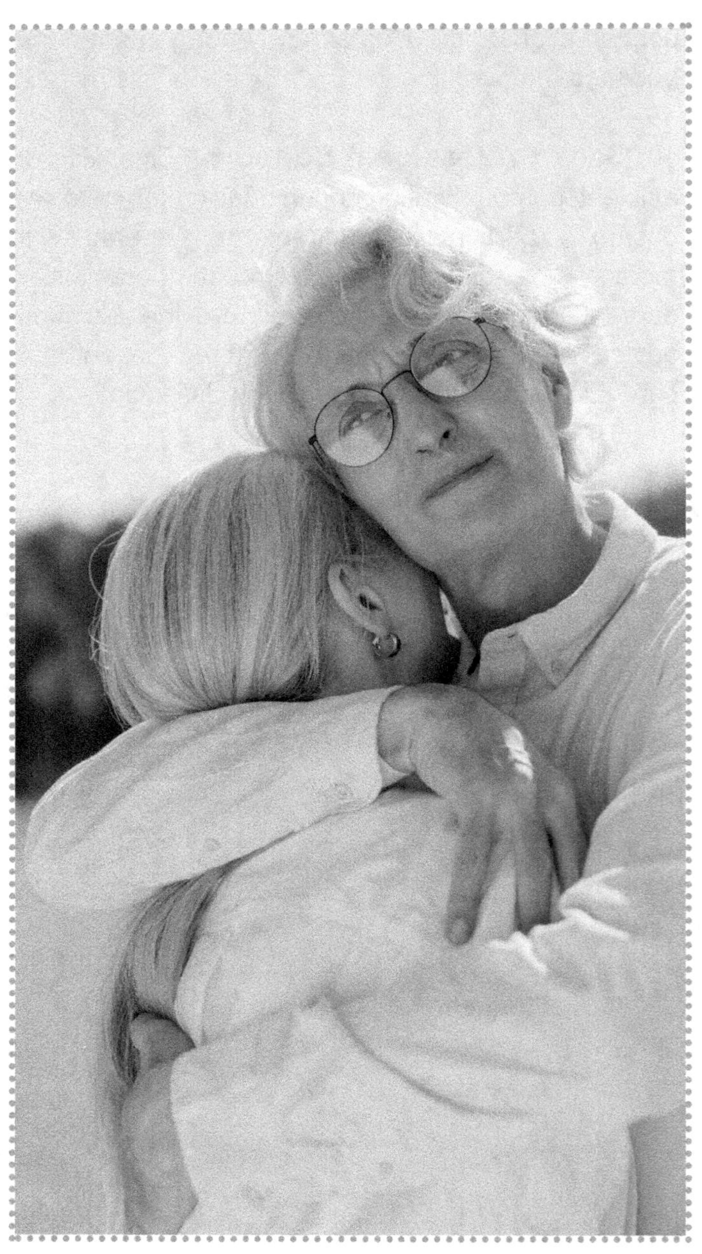

CHAPTER THREE

Memory-Boosting Activities

Millions of people worldwide suffer from dementia, a difficult illness that impairs memory, cognition, and day-to-day functioning. Dementia does not currently have a cure, but there are a number of techniques and pursuits that can lessen its effects and enhance quality of life in general. Therefore, we will examine two crucial strategies for improving the victim's cognitive function.

Reminiscence therapy:

Oftentimes, structured activities are used to help people recall past experiences, events, and memories. For dementia patients, this therapeutic approach has demonstrated encouraging outcomes in terms of mood, cognitive function, and general quality of life. The following list of memory exercises is specifically designed for people with dementia:

1. **Memory Scrapbooking**: - Give scrapbooking supplies, pictures, and mementos to patients who are suffering from dementia.

- Inspire them to compile scrapbooks or memory albums that highlight important occasions, locations, and figures from their history.
Lead them through the procedure, asking them to recollections and tales connected to every object they add. This exercise improves self-expression and creativity in addition to memory.

2. **Life Review Sessions**: - Set up individual or group sessions where people with dementia can consider various phases of their lives.

- To spark memories and promote conversation, use cues like music, historical events, or old newspapers.

- Create a welcoming space for patients to talk about their experiences, successes, and struggles.

- Lead meaningful discussions that affirm their experiences and offer chances for them to express and connect their emotions.

3. **Activities for Sensory Stimulation**: - Involve dementia patients in sensory-based memory exercises, like music therapy, aromatherapy, or tactile stimulation.

- To arouse feelings and memories, use smells, music, and textures from their past.

Add objects from their childhood that they are familiar with, vintage clothing, or old-fashioned candies to improve the sensory experience. These pursuits have the capacity to arouse strong feelings and memories, offering an abundance of material for reflection.

4. **Virtual Reality Reminiscence**: - Make use of virtual reality technology to bring historical environments and events back to life.

- Give dementia patients virtual reality headsets loaded with immersive scenes, like old homes, historical sites, or family get-togethers.

- Permit them to explore these digital environments and engage with objects that evoke feelings and memories.

- Patients can experience a unique and powerful way to interact with their memories by traveling back in time with virtual reality reminiscence.

5. **Memory Boxes**: - Make individualized memory boxes that are stuffed with objects that are particularly meaningful to dementia patients.

- Incorporate pictures, mementos, heirlooms, and other items that bring back memories of their past.

- Urge patients to look through the items in their memory boxes and remember the memories and feelings connected to each one. A person can find comfort and a sense of connection from memory boxes, which act as tangible reminders of their past, even in the face of dementia's challenges.

Memory Games and Exercises:

Playing memory games and exercises with dementia patients can help stimulate cognitive function, improve attention and concentration, and foster mental agility in addition to reminiscence therapy. The following list of memory-enhancing activities is specific to those with dementia:

1. **Word Games**: Word games are a great way to improve vocabulary and language skills. Examples of these games include crossword puzzles, word searches, and word association exercises.

- To take different levels of cognitive ability into account, select puzzles with varying degrees of difficulty.

When support and motivation are required, give it, keeping in mind the process above the result.

2. **Number Games**: - Mathematical reasoning and problem-solving abilities can be enhanced by number-based games such as Sudoku, math puzzles, and counting exercises.

- As patients gain proficiency, start with simpler puzzles and progressively increase the complexity.
- Use real-world examples and useful math applications to add relevance and interest to the activities.

3. **Memory Matching Games**: Memory matching games, sometimes called pairs or concentration games, require players to match images or cards in pairs.

- Make use of cards with well-known images, phrases, or symbols that are associated with the hobbies and experiences of the patient.

- Start with fewer cards and add more pairs to progressively increase the difficulty.

- Playing this game enhances focus, visual memory, and attention to detail.

4. **Trivia Quizzes**: - Create trivia questions on a variety of subjects, such as pop culture, music, literature, history, and pop culture.
Make sure the patient feels challenged and involved by customizing the questions to their interests and level of knowledge.

- To foster camaraderie and social interaction, encourage friendly competition and group participation.

- Trivia tests are a fun method to assess general knowledge and memory recall while enhancing cognitive function.

5. **Exercises for Sensory Stimulation**: - Give dementia patients sensory-based activities that aim to stimulate various senses and improve memory retrieval.

- Reminiscences and feelings can be evoked by engaging in activities like indulging in flavors, smelling familiar scents, or listening to music from their youth.

- Invite patients to talk about the memories and stories that go along with their sensory experiences.

- Exercises that stimulate multiple neural pathways and foster cognitive engagement offer a multisensory approach to memory improvement.

Results showed that Including memory games and exercises and reminiscence therapy in dementia care programs can significantly improve patients' mental health, cognitive function, and general quality of life. These exercises give patients worthwhile chances to interact with their recollections, sharpen their cognitive abilities, and strengthen their social ties. Caregivers can design individualized interventions that support cognitive health and improve the quality of life for dementia patients by customizing activities to each patient's preferences and abilities.

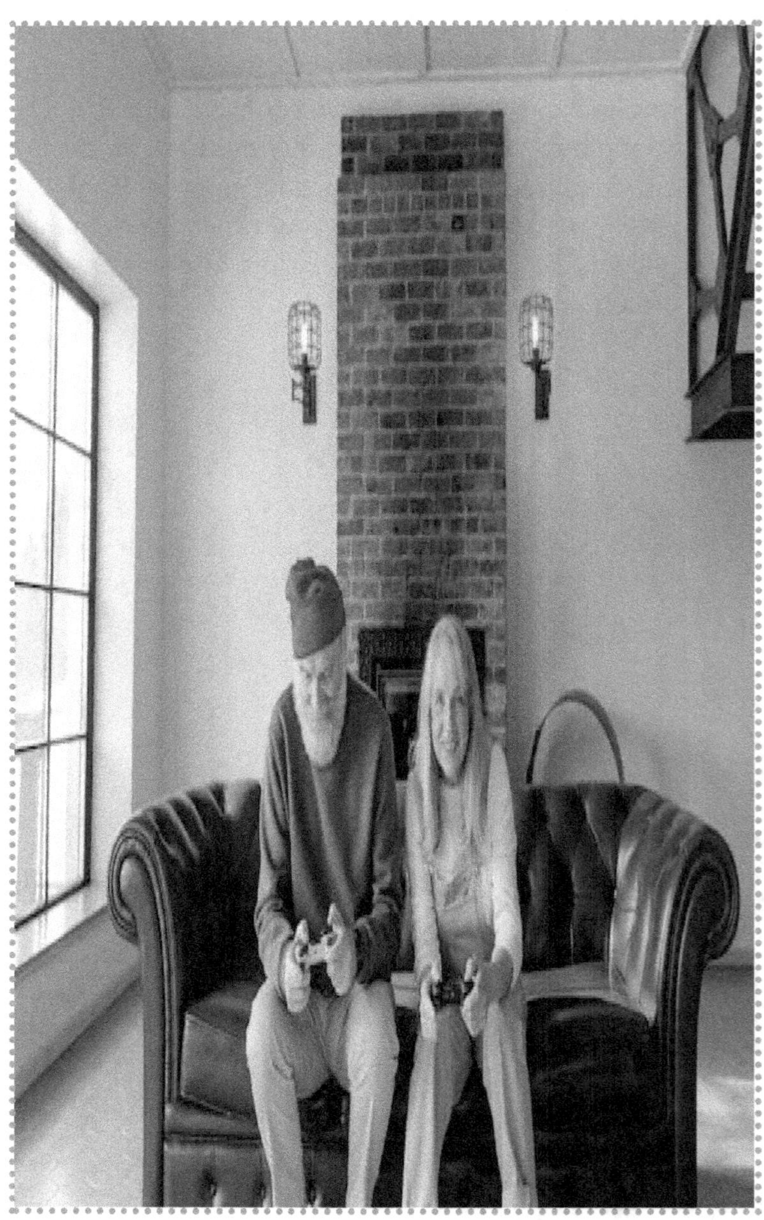

CHAPTER FOUR

Exploring the World of Sensory Stimulation

Within the human experience, sensory stimulation is essential in forming our thoughts, feelings, and general state of health. Our senses are in constant contact with the environment around us, taking in everything from the fragrance of newly opened flowers to the warmth of sunlight on our skin. Professionals from a wide range of disciplines have embraced the idea of multi-sensory environments and activities as a way to improve quality of life, encourage relaxation, and foster cognitive development because they understand the profound impact of sensory experiences. Among these creative strategies, sensory gardens stick out as immersive environments created to stimulate the senses and promote overall wellbeing. We explore the fascinating field of sensory stimulation in this investigation, learning the value of multisensory activities and the potential therapeutic benefits of sensory gardens and environments.

The Importance of Sensory Stimulation:

The activation of the senses by a variety of stimuli, such as sight, sound, touch, taste, and smell, is referred to as sensory stimulation. These sensory inputs impact our mood, cognitive function, and overall sensory processing, all of which are important for how we view and engage with our environment. In particular, sensory stimulation can help improve sensory integration, lower anxiety, and improve communication skills in people with sensory processing disorders, such as dementia or autism spectrum disorder.

Multi-Senses Involved

Multimodal activities comprise an extensive array of interactive experiences intended to stimulate multiple senses concurrently. These exercises are adaptable, making them useful resources for therapy, education, and leisure across a range of age groups, skills, and interests. Multisensory activities help kids develop their social skills, cognitive abilities, and sensorimotor abilities. Rich sensory experiences can be provided while fostering creativity and exploration through easy activities like finger painting, music and movement sessions, or sensory bins filled with different textures.

Multisensory activities are used in therapeutic settings to target particular sensory needs and encourage arousal control or relaxation. To assist clients who struggle with sensory processing to learn adaptive responses to stimuli, occupational therapists frequently include sensory-rich environments and activities into their sessions. For those who struggle with sensory modulation, deep pressure activities like vibrating cushions or weighted blankets can offer soothing sensory input.

A Sanctuary for the Senses [Sensory Gardens]

A special fusion of the natural world's beauty and sensory stimulation can be found in sensory gardens, which create immersive settings that captivate guests on several levels. These thoughtfully chosen areas are meant to stimulate the senses, elicit feelings, and encourage rest and wellbeing.

A sensory garden allows guests to enjoy the tactile pleasure of running their fingers through soft foliage, the calming sounds of trickling water or rustling leaves, the fragrant scents of herbs and spices, and the brilliant colors of blooming flowers.

Sensual gardens are more than just beautiful landscapes; they are healing spaces for people of all ages and abilities. Sensory gardens offer beneficial chances for sensory integration and exploration in a realistic environment for kids with sensory processing disorders. Diverse sensory needs and preferences are catered to by interactive elements like raised garden beds for tactile gardening activities, sensory pathways with varying textures beneathfoot, and wind chimes.

The therapeutic benefits of sensory gardens in promoting relaxation, lowering stress levels, and improving general well-being are becoming more widely acknowledged in healthcare settings. According to research, spending time in natural settings can improve psychological and physiological health. These benefits include lowered blood pressure, happier moods, and greater feelings of calm and connection to the natural world.

Building Sensation-Rich Spaces

It is important to carefully consider a number of factors when designing environments that are rich in sensory experiences, such as sensory preferences, accessibility, safety, and aesthetic appeal. To meet the needs and preferences of each sense, sensory environments—whether they are indoors or outdoors—should provide a harmony of invigorating and soothing elements.

A range of sensory stimuli, including tactile, olfactory, visual, auditory, and proprioceptive experiences, should be included to enable people to interact meaningfully with their surroundings. For instance, a sensory room in a medical facility might have tactile surfaces, cozy seating, relaxing music, and soft lighting to promote relaxation and sensory exploration.

When creating sensory environments, accessibility is a crucial factor to take into account, especially for people who have mobility or sensory impairments. Ensuring everyone can fully participate and benefit from the sensory experience is ensured by providing wheelchair-accessible pathways, tactile signage, and adjustable sensory equipment.

In brief:
A vital component of the human experience, sensory stimulation affects our perceptions, feelings, and general wellbeing. People of all ages and abilities can interact meaningfully with the world, supporting cognitive development, encouraging relaxation, and improving quality of life, through multisensory activities and environments. Specifically, sensory gardens provide immersive sanctuaries where guests can experience the wonders of nature while their

senses are piqued and their souls are fed. We can unleash the transformative power of sensory stimulation and create more enriching experiences for everyone by adopting the principles of sensory integration and building inclusive, sensory-rich environments.

CHAPTER FIVE

Nurturing the Mind and Soul

[Creative Expressions and Therapies
for Individuals Living with Dementia]

Dementia affects memory, cognitive function, and emotional well-being, posing serious challenges to both the affected person and their loved ones. When it gets harder for people with dementia to communicate and express themselves through traditional means, creative therapies provide important ways for them to interact with the outside world, express their feelings, and connect with their inner selves. In this investigation, we examine the ways that creative expressions, such as music therapy, movement therapy, and art therapy, can improve the quality of life for dementia patients.

Revealing the Inner Canvas through Art Therapy

Through nonverbal communication, art therapy helps people communicate beyond cognitive and linguistic barriers. People with dementia can access their inner creativity, memories, and emotions by creating art in various media such as painting, drawing, and sculpture. Through art therapy, people can express themselves in a secure and encouraging setting and share ideas and emotions that they might find challenging to express verbally.

Art therapy can act as a cognitive stimulant for people who are in the early stages of dementia, preserving cognitive function and a sense of identity and purpose. Easy art projects that build self-esteem and a sense of accomplishment include finger painting, collage, and memory boxes. Art therapy can be a comforting and emotional release for people with dementia as their condition worsens, enabling them to process complex emotions like grief and frustration.

Furthermore, the act of creating itself can be therapeutic, giving one a sense of empowerment and control in an increasingly chaotic and uncertain world. Regardless of the result, people with dementia can find comfort and joy in the act of creating by paying attention to the present and partaking in sensory experiences.

Harmonies for Soul Healing through Music Therapy

The brain is profoundly affected by music, which stimulates neural pathways, evokes memories, and elicits emotional responses. Through the therapeutic benefits of music, music therapy helps people with dementia function better cognitively, feel better emotionally, and live better overall. Music therapy is a multimodal experience that uses singing, playing instruments, or listening to engage people on a deep emotional level.

The power of music therapy to access memories and emotions that might otherwise be unreachable owing to cognitive decline is one of its most amazing features. Well-known songs from their past can bring back memories of important occasions, connections, and intimate moments, strengthening their sense of identity and connection to the world. People with dementia can experience the joy of creating music in group music therapy sessions, which fosters social interactions and a sense of community. Apart from its advantageous effects on cognition and emotions, music therapy can also tackle the physical manifestations of dementia, like restlessness, fear, and insomnia. Relaxing music can help people unwind and feel less stressed, and rhythmic exercises like dancing or drumming can enhance their balance and motor coordination.

Embodying the Rhythm of Life through Movement Therapy

Rhythmic movement exercises, dance, yoga, tai chi, and other physical activities are all included in movement therapy, which aims to improve mental, emotional, and physical health. Movement therapy provides a comprehensive approach to care that acknowledges the interdependence of the mind, body, and spirit for people with dementia.

Particularly dance therapy has been demonstrated to be extremely helpful for people with dementia, offering them a creative outlet for self-expression, social interaction, and physical activity. People can express their emotions, connect with others, and discover the possibilities of their bodies in a safe and encouraging setting by participating in improvisational dance and guided movement exercises.

For those suffering from dementia, yoga and tai chi, which emphasize mindful movement, breathing exercises, and mild stretching, can be especially beneficial as they promote relaxation, flexibility, and better balance. These age-old techniques encourage awareness and present-moment living, which supports people in developing inner serenity and fortitude in the face of cognitive difficulties.

In brief;
When it comes to helping people with dementia connect with themselves, express their feelings, and interact with the world around them, creative expression and therapy are invaluable resources. These all-encompassing approaches—whether via music therapy, art therapy, or movement therapy—address the various needs of people suffering from dementia while enhancing cognitive function, emotional stability, and general quality of life. We can improve the lives of those impacted by dementia and help them feel like they have a purpose, dignity, and a sense of belonging by appreciating the transformative power of creativity and each person's unique strengths and abilities.

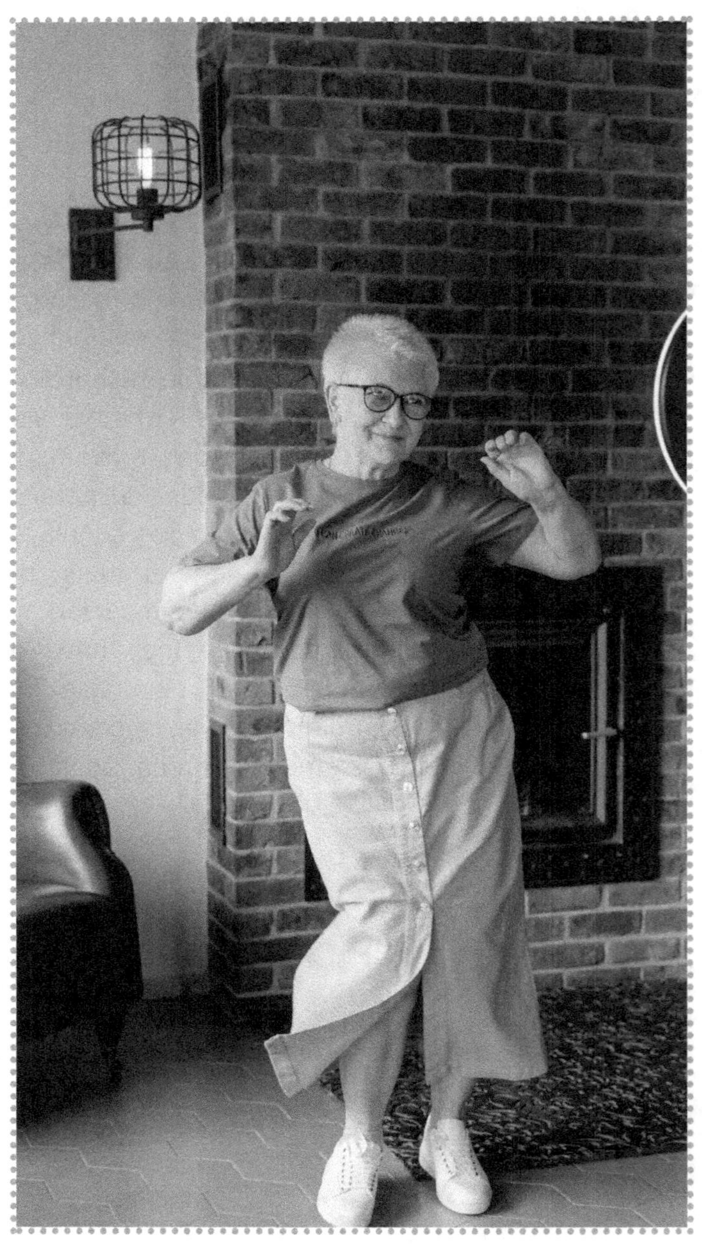

CHAPTER SIX

Mindfulness and Relaxation

Dementia patients and their caregivers face particular challenges when living with the disease. Even though the illness may affect memory and cognitive function, incorporating mindfulness and relaxation practices into daily life can have a number of positive effects, such as lowering stress levels, boosting emotional health, and enhancing general quality of life. We will examine how mindfulness, relaxation, mindful meditation, and particular relaxation techniques can be tailored to support people with dementia in this extensive guide.

Awareness of Dementia and Its Difficulties

A progressive neurological disorder called dementia is typified by a loss of cognitive abilities, such as judgment, memory, language, and problem-solving techniques. While Lewy body dementia and vascular dementia are two other types of dementia, Alzheimer's disease is the most prevalent kind.

The symptoms of dementia in people can be extremely upsetting and overwhelming. Increased agitation, confusion, and anxiety are possible, especially in new or stimulating environments. Frustration and a sense of being in the dark can also result from memory and cognitive changes.

Advantages of Relaxation and Mindfulness for Individuals with Dementia

Although there is presently no treatment for dementia, adopting mindfulness and relaxation practices into daily life can help lessen some of the psychological and emotional symptoms that are connected to the illness. Among the main advantages are:

1. **Stress Reduction**: By lowering stress levels, mindfulness and relaxation methods can improve dementia patients' feelings of peace and wellbeing.

2. **Emotional Regulation**: Through mindfulness training, people with dementia can learn to better control their emotions, which will lessen their frustration, agitation, and anxiety.

3. **Improved Quality of Life**: Mindfulness and relaxation exercises can improve dementia patients' general quality of life by encouraging a stronger sense of contentment and serenity.

4. **Enhanced Communication**: By promoting more meaningful interactions and connections, mindfulness techniques can help dementia patients and their caregivers communicate more effectively.

5. **Increased Engagement**: By giving dementia patients opportunities to participate in pleasurable and stimulating experiences, mindfulness exercises and relaxation techniques help them feel more fulfilled and purposeful.

Achievable Calming Methods for Individuals with Dementia

It's crucial to select simple, pleasurable activities that fit each dementia patient's unique preferences and abilities when implementing relaxation techniques for them. The following are some useful relaxation methods that can be modified for people suffering from dementia:

1. **Soft Breathing Techniques**: Easy breathing techniques can ease tension and encourage relaxation. Breathe deeply through your nose and slowly out of your mouth to promote slow, deep

breathing. The rhythm of the breath can also be guided by visual cues, like holding a feather or blowing bubbles.

2. **Gentle Movement Activities**: Make time each day for gentle movement exercises like Tai Chi or chair yoga. These exercises don't involve a lot of physical effort and instead encourage body awareness, flexibility, and relaxation.

5. **Nature Exposure**: Being outside in nature can help to relax the body and mind. Sit outside and take in the sights and sounds of nature, or stroll leisurely through a garden or park. Urge the person to use all of their senses, taking in the sights, sounds, and smells of their environment.

Meditative Practices for Individuals with Dementia

There are modified mindfulness techniques that can be tailored to the needs and abilities of individuals with advanced dementia, even though traditional meditation practices may present difficulties for them. With dementia patients, mindful meditation can be done in the following ways:

1. **Guided Imagery**: Guide the person through relaxing visualizations using scripts or recordings for guided imagery. Select straightforward, relatable, and captivating imagery, like picturing a calm beach or serene forest. Urge the person to fully immerse themselves in the experience by encouraging them to use their senses.

2. **Breath Awareness**: Assist the person in focusing on their breathing while performing basic breath awareness exercises. Help them connect with their breathing rhythm by using tactile or visual cues, like blowing bubbles or placing a hand on the abdomen. Urge them to pay attention to how their breath feels as it enters and exits their body.

3. **Sensory Meditation**: Investigate various sensory experiences to awaken the person's senses in mindful meditation. Give them a range of textured items, like silky textiles or polished stones, to touch and investigate mindfully, for instance. Invite them to describe their feelings without passing judgment.

4. **Meditation on Loving-Kindness**: In order to practice loving-kindness meditation, assist the person in developing compassion and kindness toward both themselves and other people. Suggest them to repeat simple affirmations, like "May I be happy, may I be healthy, may I be at peace," either aloud or silently.

5. **Nature Meditation**: Incorporate sounds of the natural world, like birdsong or running water, into your meditation sessions. Urge the person to close their eyes and visualize being in a serene outdoor environment with all the sights, sounds, and scents of nature.

Including Calm and Mindfulness in Everyday Care

The well-being of dementia patients can be significantly improved by incorporating mindfulness and relaxation techniques into regular care routines. To incorporate these practices into providing care, consider the following advice:

1. **Create a Calming Environment**: Prepare the ground for relaxation by establishing a distraction-free, peaceful, and tranquil setting. Reduce the amount of noise and clutter in the space, dim the lights, and turn on some relaxing music.

2. **Create Regular Routines** : Create dependable schedules that include relaxation techniques at regular times during the day. For dementia patients, consistency and predictability can lessen anxiety and increase a sense of security.

3. **Be Present and Patient**: Focus on being totally present in the moment with the person receiving care, approaching the task with patience and mindfulness. In your interactions, engage in active listening, show empathy and compassion, and give activities and transitions plenty of time.

4. **Offer Choices and Encouragement**: Give the person the power to take charge of their own care by providing them with options and chances for independence. Give them the freedom to make decisions and encourage them to partake in meaningful and pleasurable leisure activities.

5. **Practice Self-Care**: As a caregiver, never forget to put your own health first. Take up self-care and relaxation exercises to control your stress and avoid burnout. Taking care of yourself makes it easier for you to meet the needs of the dementia patient.

To sum up, mindfulness and relaxation methods are useful resources for helping people who are suffering from dementia. You can support patients and caregivers in feeling more at ease, connected, and well-being by implementing these practices into daily life and caregiving routines. Always remember to treat each interaction with the person who has dementia with patience, compassion, and mindfulness, respecting their individual needs and abilities. With regular practice and a nurturing atmosphere, mindfulness and relaxation can develop into effective tools for improving life quality and creating peaceful moments even in the face of dementia's challenges.

CHAPTER SEVEN

Physical Activities and Gentle Exercises

Seniors' general health and wellbeing, especially that of those suffering from dementia or Alzheimer's disease, depend heavily on continuing their physical activity and exercise. Adapting physical activities to their abilities can offer many benefits, including improved mobility, balance, mood, and cognitive function, even though cognitive decline may present challenges. We will examine mild exercises and modified physical activities created especially for elderly people with dementia in this thorough guide, enabling them to remain active and involved in meaningful ways.

Numerous advantages of physical activity for people with dementia have been demonstrated, including:

1. **Enhanced Mobility and Functionality**: Regular exercise helps preserve joint mobility, muscle strength, and flexibility, which encourages independence in day-to-day tasks.

2. **Better Mood and Well-Being**: Exercise releases endorphins, which are the body's natural feel-good hormones. These hormones can lift your spirits, lessen anxiety and depression, and make you feel better all around.

3. **Better Sleep Quality**: Getting regular exercise helps lengthen and enhance sleep, which lowers the likelihood of sleep disturbances that are frequently linked to dementia.

4. **Cognitive Benefits**: Research has demonstrated that exercise supports cognitive function and may help dementia patients delay the onset of cognitive decline.

Modifying Exercise

It's critical to take into account each senior's unique abilities, interests, and preferences when creating physical activities for those with dementia. The following are some fundamental ideas for modifying physical activities:

1. **Keep it Simple**: Select simple tasks that need little guidance and are easily understood. Exercises should be broken down into manageable steps with precise instructions.

2. **Put the Fun First**: Give top priority to pursuits that make each person happy and engaged. When choosing activities, take into account their interests, hobbies, and prior experiences.

3. **Promote Safety**: Make sure that there are no risks present, such as sharp objects or slick floors. Keep a close eye on things to avoid mishaps or injuries.

4. **Offer Support and Encouragement**: Throughout the exercise, offer support and encouragement. Provide support when required, but let the person take part at their own leisure.

5. **Be Flexible and Easy**: Be ready to modify tasks in accordance with each person's requirements and capacity. Be patient, adaptable, and open to changing activities as needed during each session.

Silent Activities for Elderly People with Dementia

Here are some gentle exercises specifically tailored for seniors with dementia:

1. **Seated Exercises**: Seated exercises are ideal for seniors with limited mobility or balance issues. These exercises can be performed while sitting in a

chair or wheelchair and focus on improving strength, flexibility, and circulation. Examples include seated leg lifts, arm curls with light weights, and seated marching.

2. **Gentle Stretching**: Gentle stretching exercises help maintain flexibility and range of motion in the joints. Encourage the individual to perform simple stretches targeting major muscle groups, such as the shoulders, arms, legs, and neck. For ten to thirty seconds, hold each stretch, then repeat as necessary.

3. **Balance Exercises**: Improving stability and reducing the risk of falls are two benefits of balance exercises. Easy balance drills that can be tailored to the person's abilities include walking heel to toe or standing on one leg. When necessary, provide stability by using a countertop or strong chair as support.

4. **Tai Chi and Qigong**: Tai Chi and Qigong are low-impact, gentle forms of exercise with an emphasis on deep breathing and slow, flowing movements. Balance, coordination, and relaxation can all be enhanced by these mind-body techniques. Make the movements simple and straightforward, with an emphasis on mindful breathing and soft, flowing motions.

5. **Chair Yoga**: This style of yoga modifies standard poses so they can be done sitting down or with the assistance of a chair. Stress reduction, strength, and flexibility can all be enhanced with mild stretching, breathing exercises, and relaxation methods. Concentrate on basic sitting poses like side stretches, seated forward bends, and mild twists.

Incorporating Daily Drills in our everyday life

Seniors with dementia can maintain their level of activity and engagement by incorporating physical activity into their daily routine. The following advice can help you incorporate exercise into your regular routine:

1. **Morning Movement Routine**: To awaken the body and encourage circulation, begin your day with a brief morning movement routine. This can be doing some light stretching, sitting, or taking a quick stroll around the house or yard.

2. **Active Leisure Activities**: Promote gardening, dancing, or playing easy games like bean bag toss or balloon volleyball as examples of active leisure activities that encourage movement and engagement.

3. **Regular Walks**: Depending on the person's mobility and preferences, go for regular walks with them—either indoors or outdoors. Stimulating the senses, encouraging physical activity, and taking in the outdoors can all be accomplished through walking.

4. **Dance Therapy**: Include dance and music in everyday activities to encourage emotional expression, coordination, and movement. For those suffering from dementia, dance therapy exercises like rhythmic movement or group dancing can be entertaining and engaging.

5. **Household Chores**: Assist the person with minor housework or activities that encourage mobility and self-sufficiency, like laying the table, folding clothes, or sweeping the floor. Concentrate on tasks that are appropriate for their skill level and have meaning.

Results

Exercise and physical activity are essential for maintaining the health and wellbeing of seniors, especially those who have dementia or Alzheimer's disease. People with dementia can gain many advantages from modifying physical activities to fit their preferences and abilities, such as enhanced mobility, mood, and cognitive function. Incorporating mind-body techniques like chair yoga and Tai Chi, as well as gentle stretching and seated exercises, can improve overall quality of life and support both physical and emotional well-being. Keep in mind to respect the individual with dementia's particular needs and abilities by approaching each activity with patience, adaptability, and an emphasis on enjoyment. Seniors with dementia can retain their independence, dignity, and sense of purpose as they move through life by regularly participating in physical activity.

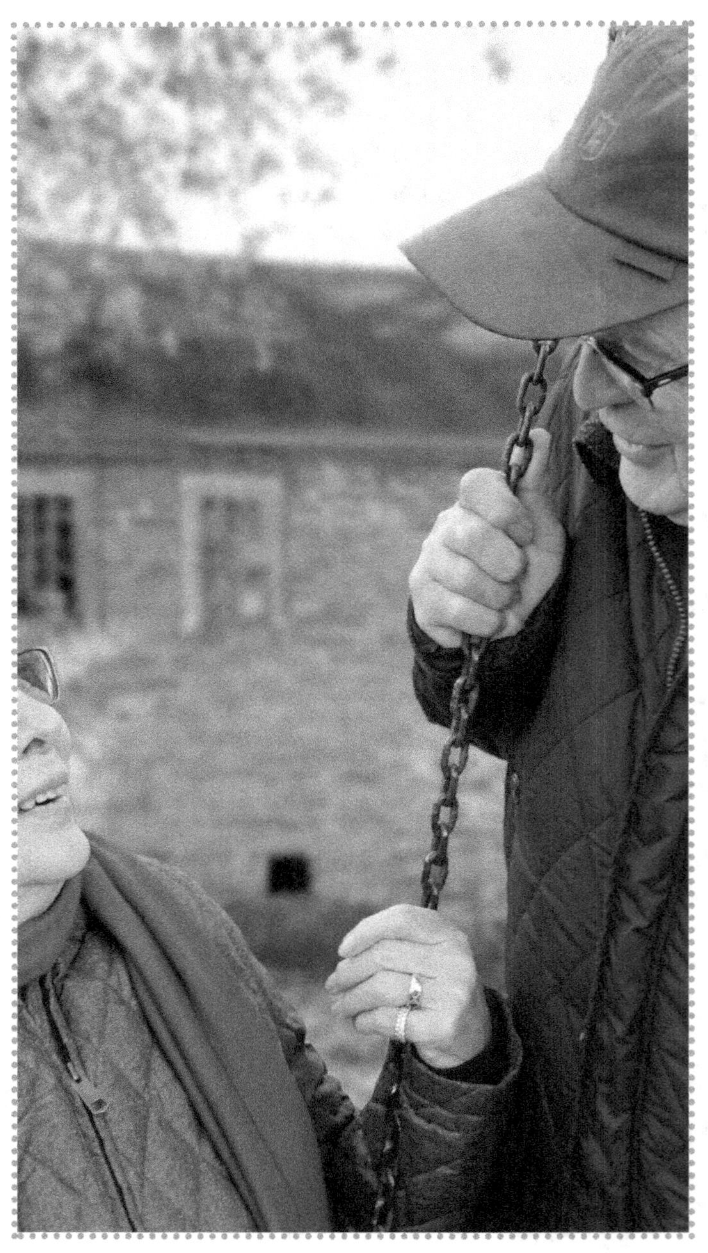

CHAPTER EIGHT

Cognitive Stimulation

[Enhancing Mental Well-being]

People with dementia face many difficulties because the condition gradually impairs their memory, cognitive function, and general mental health. Nonetheless, there are numerous approaches to help dementia patients' cognitive health and mind stimulation. Engaging and enjoyable opportunities to exercise the brain, promote mental agility and improve overall well-being are provided by cognitive stimulation activities. We'll examine the value of cognitive stimulation for dementia patients in this guide, along with games, puzzles, and cognitive challenges that are specially designed to meet their needs.

Understanding Cognitive Stimulation

Cognitive stimulation involves engaging in activities and exercises designed to challenge and stimulate the brain. These activities aim to maintain cognitive function, encourage neural plasticity, and improve mental resilience. For dementia patients, cognitive stimulation is particularly important as it can help slow cognitive decline, reduce feelings of frustration, and enhance quality of life.

Benefits of Cognitive Stimulation for Dementia Patients

Engaging in regular cognitive stimulation activities offers numerous benefits for dementia patients:

1. **Preserving Cognitive Function**: Cognitive stimulation can help slow down the rate of cognitive decline, preserving memory, reasoning, and problem-solving abilities for longer periods.

2. **Improving Mood**: Participating in stimulating activities can boost mood and emotional well-being, reducing feelings of depression, anxiety, and agitation commonly experienced by dementia patients.

3. **Enhancing Social Interaction**: Many cognitive stimulation activities are group-based, providing opportunities for social interaction, engagement, and connection with others, which is essential for mental and emotional health.

4. **Increasing Confidence**: Successfully completing cognitive challenges and puzzles can boost confidence and self-esteem in dementia patients, fostering a sense of accomplishment and empowerment.

5. **Promoting Brain Health**: Cognitive stimulation activities promote brain health by stimulating neural pathways, encouraging the formation of new connections, and supporting overall cognitive resilience.

Brain Training Games for Dementia Patients

Brain training games are specifically designed to target various cognitive functions, including memory, attention, language, and executive function. These games offer enjoyable and accessible ways to challenge the brain and promote mental sharpness in dementia patients. Here are some brain traning games suitable for dementia patients:

1. **Memory Games**: Memory games, such as matching pairs, memory cards, and recall exercises, are excellent for stimulating memory function in dementia patients. These games can be adapted to suit different ability levels and preferences.

2. **Word Games**: Word games, such as crossword puzzles, word searches, and vocabulary quizzes, help improve language skills and promote word recall in dementia patients. Choose games with

clear and simple instructions to maximize accessibility.

3. **Logic Puzzles**: Logic puzzles, such as Sudoku, logic grids, and cryptograms, challenge cognitive flexibility, problem-solving skills, and logical reasoning abilities in dementia patients. Start with simpler puzzles and gradually increase the difficulty level as skills improve.

4. **Pattern Recognition**: Pattern recognition games, such as jigsaw puzzles, visual matching tasks, and sequence completion exercises, enhance visual-spatial skills and promote cognitive processing speed in dementia patients.

5. **Numeracy Challenges**: Numeracy challenges, such as simple calculations, number sequencing, and counting exercises, help maintain numeracy skills and promote mental arithmetic in dementia patients.

Cognitive-Challenges,and Puzzles for the victims

In addition to brain training games, a variety of cognitive challenges and puzzles can provide stimulating mental activity for dementia patients. These challenges engage different cognitive abilities and offer opportunities for creativity, problem-solving, and critical thinking. Here are some examples of cognitive challenges and puzzles suitable for dementia patients:

1. **Creative Expression**: Encourage dementia patients to engage in creative activities, such as drawing, painting, coloring, or crafting. These activities stimulate imagination, promote self-expression, and provide a therapeutic outlet for emotional expression.

2. **Reminiscence Therapy**: Reminiscence therapy involves stimulating memories and engaging in meaningful conversations about past experiences, events, and personal stories. Use photographs, music, and other sensory cues to trigger memories and facilitate reminiscence sessions.

3. **Trivia and Quizzes**: Host trivia sessions or quiz games focused on topics of interest to the dementia patient, such as history, geography, or popular culture. Trivia games stimulate memory recall, promote social interaction, and provide opportunities for learning and reminiscing.

4. **Problem Solving Activities**: Problem-solving activities, such as riddles, logic puzzles, and brainteasers, challenge cognitive flexibility, reasoning, and critical thinking skills in dementia patients. Encourage creative thinking and experimentation to solve the puzzles.

5. **Adapted Board Games**: Modify traditional board games, such as chess, checkers, or Scrabble, to make them more accessible for dementia patients. Simplify rules, provide visual cues, and offer assistance as needed to ensure an enjoyable and engaging experience.

Incorporating Cognitive Stimulation into Daily Routine

Incorporating cognitive stimulation activities into the daily routine of dementia patients requires creativity, patience, and flexibility. Here are some practical tips for caregivers and healthcare professionals:

1. **Personalize Activities**: Tailor cognitive stimulation activities to suit the individual preferences, interests, and abilities of the dementia patient. Consider their past hobbies, occupations, and life experiences when selecting activities.

2. **Provide Support and Guidance**: Offer encouragement, support, and guidance to dementia patients as they engage in cognitive stimulation activities. Break tasks into manageable steps, provide cues and prompts as needed, and celebrate small achievements.

3. **Create a Stimulating Environment**: Establish a stimulating environment that encourages engagement and participation in cognitive stimulation activities. Use bright colors, familiar objects, and comfortable seating arrangements to make the space inviting and accessible.

4. **Maintain a Routine**: Establish a consistent daily routine that includes dedicated time for cognitive stimulation activities. Consistency and predictability help dementia patients feel more comfortable and engaged in the activities.

5. **Be Calm and Flexible****: Approach cognitive stimulation activities with patience, flexibility, and a positive attitude. Recognize that progress may be gradual, and be open to adapting activities based on the individual's changing needs and abilities.

6. **Encourage Social Interaction**: Many cognitive stimulation activities can be done in group settings, providing opportunities for social interaction, engagement, and connection with others. Encourage participation in group activities to foster a sense of community and belonging.

7. **Monitor Progress and Adjust**: Monitor the progress of dementia patients as they engage in cognitive stimulation activities and adjust the activities accordingly. Be observant of signs of

frustration or fatigue, and modify activities as needed to ensure a positive and enjoyable experience.

CHAPTER NINE

Caregiver Support and Resources:

[Empowering Caregivers for the Journey]

Caring for a loved one with dementia can be a challenging and emotionally taxing experience. Caregivers often face a range of physical, emotional, and logistical challenges as they navigate the complexities of dementia care. However, caregivers are not alone in their journey. There are numerous support services, resources, and community networks available to assist and empower caregivers in providing the best possible care for their loved ones with dementia. In this comprehensive guide, we will explore caregiver support and resources, self-care strategies for caregivers, and community support networks for dementia patients and their families.

Caregiver-Support,and-Resources

Caregiver support services offer valuable assistance, guidance, and resources to caregivers of individuals living with dementia. These services aim to alleviate caregiver stress, provide practical assistance, and enhance the quality of care provided to dementia patients. Here are some common caregiver support and resources available:

1. **Support Groups**: Joining a support group for dementia caregivers can provide a sense of community, understanding, and empathy. Support groups offer opportunities to share experiences, receive emotional support, and exchange practical tips and advice with other caregivers facing similar challenges.

2. **Caregiver Education Programs**: Many organizations offer caregiver education programs and workshops designed to provide caregivers with essential knowledge and skills for managing dementia care. These programs cover topics such as communication strategies, behavior management techniques, and self-care practices.

3. **Respite Care Services**: Respite care services offer temporary relief for caregivers by providing

professional care for their loved ones with dementia. This allows caregivers to take breaks, attend appointments, run errands, or simply rest and recharge without worrying about their loved one's well-being.

4. **Home Care Assistance**: Home care agencies provide professional caregivers who offer assistance with activities of daily living, medication management, and companionship for individuals with dementia. Home care services can be tailored to meet the specific needs and preferences of both the caregiver and the care recipient.

5. **Telehealth Services**: Telehealth services, such as virtual support groups and remote counseling sessions, offer convenient and accessible support for caregivers who may have difficulty attending in-person events. Telehealth services provide opportunities for education, counseling, and emotional support from the comfort of home.

6. **Caregiver Resource Centers**: Many hospitals, clinics, and community organizations operate caregiver resource centers that offer information, referral services, and assistance with accessing local support resources. Caregiver resource centers provide a centralized hub for caregivers to access information and support tailored to their needs.

Self-Care for Caregivers

Taking care of oneself is essential for maintaining physical, emotional, and mental well-being as a caregiver. Self-care practices help prevent burnout, reduce stress, and enhance resilience, allowing caregivers to continue providing quality care for their loved ones with dementia. Here are some caregiver self-care techniques:

1. **Prioritize Your Health**: Make time for regular exercise, nutritious meals, and adequate sleep to maintain physical health and energy levels. Prioritize preventive healthcare, such as regular check-ups and screenings, to monitor your own well-being.

2. **Set Boundaries**: Establish clear boundaries around caregiving responsibilities and advocate for your own needs and limitations. Learn to say no to additional commitments or requests that may overwhelm you.

3. **Take Breaks**: Schedule regular breaks from caregiving to rest, relax, and recharge. Use respite care services, enlist the help of family and friends, or arrange for professional caregivers to provide temporary relief.

4. **Practice Stress Management**: Incorporate stress-reducing activities into your daily routine, such as deep breathing exercises, meditation,

yoga, or mindfulness practices. Find activities that help you relax and unwind, and make time for them regularly.

5. **Seek Social Support**: Maintain connections with family, friends, and support networks who can offer emotional support, practical assistance, and companionship. Share your thoughts, feelings, and caregiving experiences with trusted individuals who can offer understanding and empathy.

6. **Engage in Enjoyable Activities**: Make time for hobbies, interests, and activities that bring you joy and fulfillment. Engaging in enjoyable activities outside of caregiving can help you maintain a sense of identity, purpose, and satisfaction in life.

7. **Seek Professional Help**: If you're struggling to cope with the demands of caregiving, don't hesitate to seek professional help from a therapist, counselor, or support group facilitator. Professional support can provide valuable insights, coping strategies, and emotional validation.

Community-Support,and Resources for the victim's

Community support networks play a vital role in providing assistance, advocacy, and resources for individuals living with dementia and their families. These networks offer a range of services and programs designed to support dementia patients and their caregivers. Here are some community support and resources available:

1. **Alzheimer's Associations**: National and local Alzheimer's associations offer a wealth of resources, support services, and educational programs for individuals living with dementia and their caregivers. These organizations provide information, advocacy, and community outreach initiatives to raise awareness and support dementia care.

2.**Senior Centers**: Senior centers often offer programs, activities, and support groups specifically tailored to the needs of older adults, including those living with dementia. These centers provide opportunities for socialization, recreation, and engagement in a supportive and inclusive environment.

3. **Community Centers**: Community centers may offer dementia-friendly programs, workshops, and events aimed at raising awareness, providing

education, and fostering community support for individuals living with dementia and their families.

4.**Faith-Based Organizations**: Many faith-based organizations, such as churches, synagogues, and mosques, offer support groups, pastoral care services, and volunteer opportunities for individuals affected by dementia. These organizations provide spiritual and emotional support within a compassionate and inclusive community.

5.**Local Support Groups**: Local support groups for dementia patients and their caregivers provide opportunities for mutual support, shared experiences, and practical advice. These groups may be facilitated by healthcare professionals, community organizations, or volunteer caregivers.

6.**Community-Based-Programs**:Community-based programs, such as adult day centers, memory cafes, and dementia-friendly recreational activities, offer opportunities for socialization, engagement, and respite for individuals living with dementia and their caregivers.

7.**Legal and Financial Assistance**: Community organizations and advocacy groups may offer assistance with legal and financial matters related to dementia care, such as advance care planning, estate planning, and accessing financial assistance programs.

In conclusion, caregiver support and resources, self-care strategies, and community networks play essential roles in supporting individuals living with dementia and their caregivers. By accessing these resources and support services, caregivers can find assistance, guidance, and validation as they navigate the challenges of dementia care. Prioritizing self-care allows caregivers to maintain their own well-being while providing compassionate and effective care for their loved ones with dementia. Community support networks offer invaluable assistance, advocacy, and companionship for individuals living with dementia and their families, fostering a sense of belonging and support within the broader community. Through collaboration, education, and compassionate care, caregivers and community organizations can work together to enhance the quality of life for individuals affected by dementia.

CHAPTER TEN

Conclusion:

Recap of Key Strategies**

In conclusion, dementia, including Alzheimer's disease, presents significant challenges for individuals and their families. While there is currently no cure for dementia, there are several strategies that may help reduce the risk of developing the condition or delay its onset. Here's a recap of key strategies to avoiding dementia:

1. **Maintain a Healthy Lifestyle**: Adopting a healthy lifestyle that includes regular exercise, a balanced diet, adequate sleep, and stress management can help reduce the risk of dementia. Physical activity and healthy eating habits support brain health and cognitive function.

2. **Stay Mentally Active**: Engaging in mentally stimulating activities, such as reading, puzzles, learning new skills, and socializing, can help keep the brain active and reduce the risk of cognitive decline. Challenging the mind regularly can promote cognitive reserve and resilience.

3. **Manage Chronic Health Conditions**: Managing chronic health conditions, such as diabetes, hypertension, and high cholesterol, is essential for reducing the risk of dementia. Controlling these conditions through medication, lifestyle changes, and regular medical check-ups can help protect brain health.

4. **Protect Brain Health**: Taking steps to protect brain health, such as wearing protective headgear during sports and activities, avoiding head injuries, and practicing safe driving habits, can help reduce the risk of dementia associated with traumatic brain injury.

5. **Socialize and Stay Connected**: Maintaining social connections and staying engaged in meaningful activities can help reduce the risk of dementia. Social interaction, emotional support, and a sense of belonging contribute to overall well-being and cognitive health.

6. **Limit Alcohol Consumption and Avoid Smoking**: Limiting alcohol consumption and avoiding smoking are important for maintaining brain health and reducing the risk of dementia. Excessive alcohol consumption and smoking are associated with cognitive impairment and an increased risk of dementia.

7. **Stay Physically Active**: Regular physical activity is essential for maintaining brain health and reducing the risk of dementia. Exercise improves blood flow to the brain, promotes the growth of new brain cells, and reduces the risk of conditions that contribute to dementia, such as obesity and cardiovascular disease.

8. **Seek Medical Attention for Cognitive Changes**: If you or a loved one experiences significant changes in memory, thinking, or behavior, it's essential to seek medical attention promptly. Early diagnosis and intervention can help identify treatable causes of cognitive impairment and provide access to appropriate care and support services.

By adopting these key strategies, individuals can take proactive steps to reduce their risk of developing dementia and promote overall brain health and well-being.

Discussion and Questions on Dementia/Alzheimer's

1. What are the Early Signs and Symptoms of Dementia?

   - Dementia often begins with subtle changes in memory, thinking, or behavior. Common early signs and symptoms include forgetfulness, difficulty finding words, confusion, disorientation, and changes in mood or personality. Individuals may also experience difficulty completing familiar tasks or following conversations.

2. What Causes Dementia?

   - Dementia is caused by damage to brain cells, which affects cognitive function and memory. The most common cause of dementia is Alzheimer's disease, but other causes include vascular dementia, Lewy body dementia, frontotemporal dementia, and mixed dementia. Risk factors for dementia include age, genetics, family history, and lifestyle factors.

3. How is Dementia Diagnosed?

   - Dementia is typically diagnosed through a combination of medical history, physical examination, cognitive assessments, and laboratory tests. Imaging tests, such as MRI or CT scans, may be used to evaluate brain structure and detect abnormalities. A thorough evaluation by a medical expert is required for a precise diagnosis.

4. What Treatments are Available for Dementia?

- While there is currently no cure for dementia, treatment options focus on managing symptoms, slowing the progression of the disease, and improving quality of life. Medications, such as cholinesterase inhibitors and memantine, may help manage cognitive symptoms in some individuals. Non-pharmacological interventions, such as cognitive stimulation therapy, physical exercise, and behavioral therapy, can also be beneficial.

5. What Support Services are Available for Dementia Patients and their Caregivers?

- There are various support services available for dementia patients and their caregivers, including home care assistance, respite care services, caregiver support groups, educational programs, and community-based resources. These services offer practical assistance, emotional support, and guidance for navigating the challenges of dementia care.

6. How can Caregivers Practice Self-Care while Caring for a Loved One with Dementia?

- Caregivers can practice self-care by prioritizing their own physical, emotional, and mental well-being. Strategies include seeking social support, taking regular breaks, engaging in enjoyable activities, practicing stress management techniques, and seeking professional help when needed. Self-care is essential for preventing burnout and maintaining quality care for both the caregiver and the person with dementia.

7. What Research is Being Done to Understand and Treat Dementia?

- Researchers are actively studying the underlying causes of dementia, developing new diagnostic tools, and exploring potential treatments and interventions. Advances in neuroscience, genetics, and technology are helping to improve our understanding of dementia and develop novel therapeutic approaches. Clinical trials and research studies play a crucial role in advancing dementia research and finding effective treatments.

8. How Can Society and Communities Help People With Dementia?

- Communities and society can support individuals living with dementia by promoting dementia-friendly environments, raising awareness, reducing stigma, and providing access to supportive services and resources. Creating inclusive spaces, offering educational programs, and fostering social connections can help individuals with dementia and their families feel supported and included in their communities.

Overall, dementia is a complex and challenging condition that requires comprehensive support, understanding, and compassion from individuals, families, healthcare professionals, and society as a whole. By raising awareness, promoting early diagnosis, providing access to quality care, and supporting research efforts, we can work together to improve the lives of those affected by dementia and strive towards a future where effective treatments and interventions are available for all.